MW00625722

Sit Fit, Be Fit

How to Stay Healthy and Pain Free When You Sit All Day

Dr. Cheryl Gottesfeld, DC

Copyright © 2011
Dr. Cheryl Gottesfeld

All rights reserved. No part of this book may be reproduced in any form, except for the inclusion of brief quotations in a review, without permission in writing from the author or publisher.

Disclaimer

The information in this book is intended for educational use only and should not be construed as medical advice. You should consult with your physician before attempting any activity or making any lifestyle changes discussed in this book. Although every attempt is made to ensure the accuracy of the information presented, the author and publisher are not liable for any illness or injury that may result from attempting any activities or lifestyle changes presented in this book.

First Printing – 2011

Printed Publication ISBN: 978-0-9830049-0-5

eBook Publication ISBN: 978-0-9830049-1-2
(Kindle, nook, iBooks, ect.)

Printed in the United States by Morris Publishing®
3212 East Highway 30
Kearney, NE 68847
1-800-650-7888

Table Of Contents

1 • Introduction 1

2 • Is Sitting All Day Really Bad for Your Body? . . 3

3 • Anatomy 101 10

4 • The Top Five Desk Disasters and
    How to Correct Them 23

5 • The Daily Dozen Stretches 31

6 • Body Band Exercises 44

7 • Basic Lifestyle Enhancements 49

8 • Patients Speak 65

9 • References 67

Book Dedication

This being my first book, I have a heart full of gratitude to many people. First, I would like to thank my parents who always instilled in me the "you can do it" attitude. Next, I would like to thank the thousands of patients, over the last 20 years, who have entrusted their health in my hands. I would never have been able to write this book without you. Hence I dedicated a chapter in this book "Patients Speak" for you. Next in my list are all the staff members over the years. These handful of people over the years have been the back bone of the office. Stated in order of when they started working with me: Maria, Patricia, Diana, Mary, Jackie, Sylvia, and Lisa. Thank you so much, for so much, over the years. Lastly, I would like to thank Jesus Christ for blessing me with the gift to heal people via chiropractic care.

1

Introduction

Sit Fit, Be Fit is a stretching routine and daily habit recommendations designed to help you avoid chronic neck pain, back pain and headaches. These occur very often very often from years of prolonged sitting. Although this book was written primarily for those who work at desk jobs, the information in this book is valid for anyone who wants to improve their health and how they feel.

The stretches and workstation modifications included in this program are specially selected and designed so they can be performed within the confines of an average workspace in only a few minutes per day. Therefore people cannot say they do not have time to do them.

It is my sincere desire that there is something in this

book that will motivate you to make the changes necessary to avoid a chronic muscular skeletal condition.

I'm sure there are some people saying — Is sitting really that bad for me? Well after you read the next chapter, I believe you will come to the same conclusion as me
— yes it is!

2

Is Sitting All Day Really Bad for Your Body?

There is now a significant body of research demonstrating that sitting all day is hard on your body and can lead to headaches, neck pain and low back pain.[1-5] The reason is simply that the body was designed to move. Movement helps to keep all your joints well lubricated, your muscles well toned, and your connective tissue supple and healthy. Movement also facilitates blood flow to all of the body's tissues. This is especially true for your spinal discs.

Spinal discs are round, donut-shaped rings of fibrous cartilage located between each of the spinal vertebrae. They are what allow the spine to bend, twist, and help absorb the shock of everyday activities, such as walking and running. Because spinal discs do not have their own direct blood supply, they rely on the movement of the body to physically pump nutrient-rich fluids into the disc and waste products out. When you sit for long periods of time, your discs become dehydrated and will begin to break down.

When spinal discs break down, they often form bulges on their outer surface, much like an old tire does when it begins to break down. These bulges—called herniations—put pressure on the spinal cord, or the nerves exiting the spine, causing excruciating pain. Although there are many causes of low back pain, one common cause of severe low back pain is herniated discs in the spine. One of the most common causes of herniated discs is simply sitting too much. In fact, a study by Dr. Kelsy demon

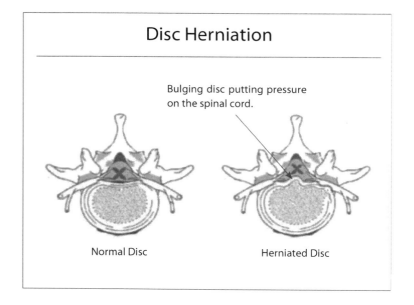

Disc Herniation

Bulging disc putting pressure on the spinal cord.

Normal Disc   Herniated Disc

strated that people who sat at their jobs more than half of their work day had a 50–60% increased risk of developing a herniated lumbar disc over those who sat less than half of the time.[6]

Another way that sitting all day leads to low back pain is that when you sit, the normal curve in your low back is flattened out. The lumbar spine is no longer in its natural lordotic (arched) position and can even become rounded when slouching. This flattening of the lumbar spine causes the ligaments in the lower back to become stretched and irritated and places undue stress on the spinal discs. A researcher by the name of Dr. Schoberth discovered that when sitting, the lumbar spine (low back) flattened out primarily at the level of the L4–L5 lumbar discs,[7] which helps to explain why low back disc herniations so commonly occur at this level.[1,3]

Prolonged sitting can also cause increased firing of the pain nerves in the lower back, resulting in low back pain. To understand why this happens, let's talk a little bit about neurology. Although there are several different types of nerves in your body, two of them are important here: those responsible for sensing pain (nociceptors), and those that help your brain keep track of your movement and posture (proprioceptors).

Whenever your body moves, your proprioceptors fire off information to your brain about what your body is doing. This allows your brain to coordinate your movements, resulting in relaxed and smooth motion. If your proprioceptors are compromised in some way—such as

The Regions of Your Spine

Cervical

Thoracic

Lumbar

Sacrum

Coccyx

Your spine is comprised of five regions. These are the cervical (neck region), the thoracic (mid back region), the lumbar (low back region), the sacrum and the Coccyx (tailbone).

occurs when the body is under the influence of alcohol—your movements and balance become uncoordinated, which is why it is so dangerous to drive after you have been drinking.

When proprioceptors are simulated, they also have the effect of blocking the signals from the pain nerves in that area. In other words, if you are experiencing pain, you can move or rub the area to stimulate the proprioceptors and the pain will decrease. This is why you rub your head when you bump it on something, or why you feel so much better after you exercise. If you sit for long periods of time and don't move much, your proprioceptors aren't stimulated. Consequently, they don't block the firing of your pain fibers and you experience pain. Over time, prolonged sitting can lead to permanent damage of the nerves, joints and connective tissues.[4,8]

The Importance of Proper Posture

One of the differences between bone and muscle is that bone is designed to support the weight of the body, but muscles are not. Muscles are designed to move your bones, but will quickly become overworked, exhausted and inflamed if they have to work all the time to hold your body up. Good posture allows the weight of your head and body to be supported by your bones, rather than your muscles, allowing you to effortlessly go through your day. However, when you have poor posture, your muscles have to do a lot of the work that your bones are supposed to do. Over time, this leads to muscles that are very tight, sore, and inflamed.

One of the most common postural problems today is forward head posture (FHP). Prolonged use of a computer and playing video games are primary causes of such a

Forward Head Posture

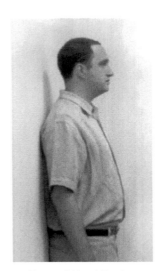 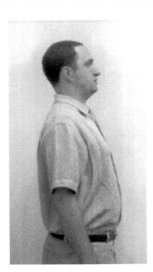

Forward Head Posture   Normal Head Posture

condition. Ideally the head should sit directly on the neck and shoulder, like a golf ball sits on a tee. The weight of your head is more like a bowling ball, weighing approximately 10 pounds. As long as the head is sitting properly over the neck and shoulders, the total stress on the spine is about ten pounds. However, if the head is translated forward, the stress on the spine is increased by ten pounds for every inch forward it is from its ideal position. According to Dr. Renee Calliet, M.D., "as the head weighing 10 lbs sits over your center, the load is only 10 lbs. However, for every inch forward your head is over your center, the weight increases by 10 lbs." Therefore, if you head is 3 inches over your shoulders, your muscles and spinal tissues are holding 30 pounds. This will eventually lead to subluxation (pinching of nerves), a loss of cervical curve and potential health problems.[9]

To illustrate this idea further, think about carrying a briefcase. If you had to carry your briefcase with your arms outstretched in front of you, it would not take long before the muscles of your shoulders would be completely exhausted. This is because carrying the briefcase far away from the center of your body places undue stress on your shoulder muscles. If you held the same briefcase down at your side, your muscles would not fatigue as quickly because the briefcase is closer to the center of your body and the weight is, therefore, supported by the bones of the skeleton, rather than the muscles.

Research performed at the Mayo clinic revealed that "FHP leads to long term muscle strain, disc herniations, arthritis and pinched nerves."[10] Additional research has shown that FHP has been shown to flatten the normal cervical curve, resulting in increased disc compression and damage and the early development of degenerative arthritis.[11]

3

Anatomy 101

Before we get into what to and how to stretch, the following is a brief overview of your basic muscular/skeletal system. The pictures in this chapter are designed to give you a visual of the muscles you will be stretching/strengthening in the chapters to follow. In this section I will be using the term "Desk Distortion Posture." This is an all-encompassing term used for poor desk posture behaviors (i.e. slouching, forward head posture, computer head, hump back . . . etc.)

The Neck

The ability of the neck is nothing short of amazing. It supports your head, which can weigh up to 16 pounds, and has an incredible range of motion. And it does all of this with only a fraction of the structural support of other areas of the spine. Unfortunately, this degree of movement coupled with limited support results in the neck being especially vulnerable to stress and strain. The muscles that are primarily affected in the neck are the trapezius, the levator scapulae and the scalenes.

The trapezius is a very large muscle which runs from the base of the skull, down to the bottom of the thoracic spine. The part of this muscle that is a problem for most people is the upper portion which runs between the base of the neck and the base of the skull. The trapezius muscle is not designed to be the primary muscle responsible for holding up the head. There are a whole host of other neck muscles which are responsible for that task. There are times when those muscles are not strong enough to keep the head up, however, and that is when the trapezius is called in to help. Unlike the normal postural muscles responsible for holding up the head, the trapezius becomes fatigued, tight and sore if it has to help out for very long, which frequently happens in people who work at desk jobs.

The second muscle that we are concerned about is the levator scapulae that runs from the upper inside tip of the shoulder blade to the base of the skull. Like the trapezius, the levator is not designed to help hold up the head for long periods of time. But also like the trapezius, the levator is frequently in a state of continual stress in those who work at desk jobs because of the Desk Distortion Posture.

The Major Muscles of the Neck

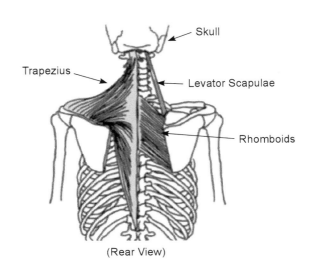

(Rear View)

The trapezius and the levator scapulae are frequently in a state of continual stress in those who work at desk jobs because of their desk distortion posture.

The third muscle of interest to us is a group of muscles called the posterior cervicals. These are the powerful muscles that run down the back of the neck and are responsible for keeping your neck straight and your head upright. The posterior cervicals lie against the spine beneath the trapezius and levator scapulae.

The stretches and exercises in the following chapters are designed to improve your posture and the muscle tone of all three of these muscles and help alleviate stress, tension or pain in the neck.

The Upper Back

The three major muscles which we are concerned with in the upper back are: the tapezius, the rhomboid and a big muscle called the latissimus dorsi. There are certainly other muscles in the upper back, but by exercising these three major muscles, problems in the other muscles tend to be minimized. In the prior section of "the neck" we discussed the trapezius muscle, however the trapezius also plays a major role with those who suffer upper back pain.

The trapezius is a very large muscle which runs from the base of the skull to the bottom of the thoracic region of the spine and across to each shoulder. This muscle covers a lot of area. The particular area of this muscle that is a problem for most people is the upper part, which runs between the lower neck, up to the base of the skull and over the shoulders. This area is often tight, sensitive to the touch and full of trigger points, or 'knots'.

There are three reasons why this happens. The first is that when you suffer from the Desk Distortion Posture your head is carried in front of your structural center. So, in order to hold your head up, the trapezius tightens up. The second reason is that when you suffer from the Desk Distortion Posture, you tend to carry your shoulders higher than they should be. The third reason is that a tight trapezius muscle causes a weakness in your rhomboid muscle, thereby allowing your shoulders to roll forward and up.

The rhomboid muscles attach to the inside edge of the

The Major Muscles of the Upper Back

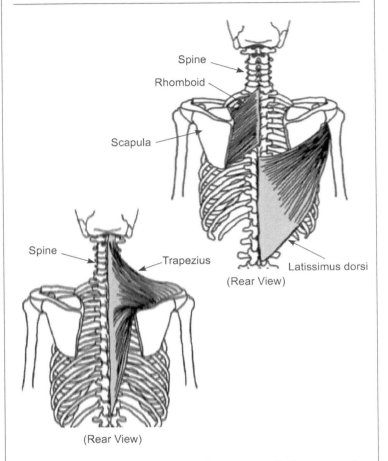

Spine

Rhomboid

Scapula

Spine

Trapezius

Latissimus dorsi

(Rear View)

(Rear View)

The three primary upper back muscles that we will discuss are the rhomboid, the latissimus dorsi, and the trapezius. People who have desk jobs will typically suffer from chronic trapezius tightness and soreness, where the rhomboid and latissimus dorsi are usually very weak. This muscular imbalance contributes to neck pain, upper back pain and headaches.

shoulder blade and run across the mid-back to the upper portion of the thoracic spine. The action of the rhomboid muscles is to pull the shoulders down and back and is just about the opposite action of the upper trapezius, which pulls the shoulders up. When the rhomboids are weak and underdeveloped, the tightness in your trapezius will tend to pull your shoulders up, thereby increasing the tension in your upper back and neck.

The latissimus dorsi muscles, also called the 'lats' for short, work with the rhomboids to pull the shoulders down and back. The difference is that the lats attach to the arm, instead of the shoulder blade where the rhomboids attach. For this reason, the lats are also very important to healthy shoulder movement.

Chest

There are two major muscle groups in the chest. These are called the pectoralis major, or simply "pec major," and the pectoralis minor, or "pec minor." In people who work at desk jobs, the pec major muscle tends to become weak from lack of use and the pec minor muscle tends to become tight due to the forward position in which the arms are held.

The pec minor, unlike the pec major, tends to go into spasm in people who work on computer or any other activity where the arms are held out in front of the body for extended periods of time. In the chapters to follow you will learn how to correct this "pec" muscular imbalance. Keeping the pec minor relaxed and flexible will help prevent chest, arm, upper back and neck pain.

The Major Muscles of the Chest

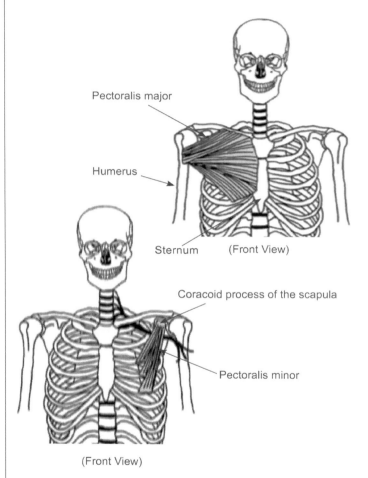

Pectoralis major

Humerus

Sternum   (Front View)

Coracoid process of the scapula

Pectoralis minor

(Front View)

The Desk Distortion Posture frequently produces tightness in the pec minor muscle. This occurs if your arms are held out in front of your body for an extended period of time.

The Low Back and Abs

The low back is by far the most frequently injured part of the body. This is due in large part to the fact that the low back, like the neck, is an unstable part of the spine, allowing us to have a lot of mobility, but at the cost of increased risk of injury. Although the low back has much more support from the muscles than the neck does, it is also exposed to dramatically more pressure and stress than the neck.

As long as all of the vertebrae in the lumbar spine are properly aligned and moving correctly and the supporting muscles are healthy and strong, the low back can withstand mind-boggling forces without injury. Professional power-lifters can pick up several hundred pounds off the floor without hurting themselves while performing a deadlift. They are able to do this because of good body mechanics – their bones and joints move correctly, their muscles are strong and coordinated, and they maintain good posture.

Those of us who work at a desk job are usually not so lucky. Because most of us sit at our job, sit while we drive to and from work and sit during much of our free time, we lose our healthy body mechanics and become much more prone to pain and injury. The Desk Distortion Posture leaves us with shortened psoas muscles, tight gluteus medius and piriformis muscles, stressed quadratus lumborum muscles and very weak abdominal muscles. Let's begin with the psoas muscle.

The psoas muscle attaches to the lowest three lumbar vertebrae, runs down through the front of the pelvis and attaches to the upper end of the femur. The psoas is a

The Low Back and Abdominals

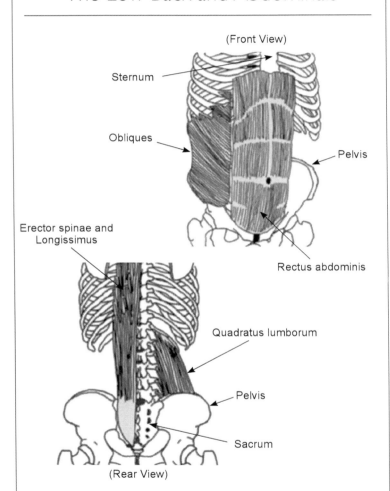

(Front View)

Sternum

Obliques

Pelvis

Erector spinae and
Longissimus

Rectus abdominis

Quadratus lumborum

Pelvis

Sacrum

(Rear View)

The four muscles that are important for low back stability are the abdominals, the obliques, the erector spinae, and the quadratus lumborum. When people sit at a desk for several hours every day, these muscles become weakened, the low back becomes unstable, and pain results.

powerful muscle which allows you to raise your upper leg. When you sit, all of the tension is taken off of the psoas muscle, allowing it to relax. If you sit for many hours every day, the lack of tension of the psoas muscle eventually causes it to shorten. The problem with shortened psoas muscles is that once you straighten your legs and stand up, they pull on the lower lumbar spine, causing back pain.

The gluteus medius and the piriformis are two muscles in the hip which can also cause problems for people who work at desk jobs. Like the psoas muscle, the gluteus medius and piriformis lose much of their flexibility and tighten up when you sit for extended periods. This muscle tightness restricts normal motion in the hip joint when you walk, but even more important is the fact that the sciatic nerve, which is the main nerve feeding the leg from the spinal cord, can become entrapped when the piriformis is tight, causing a condition called sciatica. Sciatica is a pattern of shooting pain, numbness or tingling in the leg caused by irritation of the sciatic nerve. The one way to reduce the stress on the sciatic nerve caused by pressure from a tight piriformis muscle is through exercise and stretching.

Although most people don't consider the abdominal muscles to be low back muscles, they actually are one of the most important muscle groups for stabilizing the low back. These also happen to be the least used muscles in people with desk jobs, and consequently they become very weak. The weakened abdominal muscles result in a loss of low back stability and an increased stress on the joints and other muscles, resulting in low back pain. Many people find relief from low back pain simply by ex-

Pelvis and the Low Back

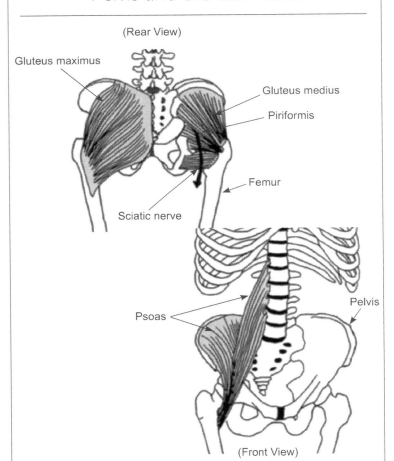

The three pelvic muscles that are of the most concern to us are the gluteus medius, the piriformis and the psoas muscles. These three muscles are important because when they are tight, they contribute to low back pain and radiating pain in the back of the legs. Due to the angle between the low back and the legs when people sit, these muscles will tighten up quickly and cause pain.

ercising and building strength in the abdominal muscles.

Two additional muscles that are a problem for people who work at jobs that require a lot of sitting are the longissimus/erector spinae group and the quadratus lumborum. The difference between these two muscles is that the quadratus lumborum is designed to be an accessory muscle for the low back and is therefore much thinner and weaker than the primary muscles of the low back; the longissimus/erector spinae group. When the low back is not exercised, the longissimus/erector spinae group becomes weaker, requiring the quadratus lumborum to pick up some of the slack. Because the quadratus lumborum muscles are not designed to do much lifting, but rather are designed to help rotate and bend the low back, this extra stress causes them to go into spasm and become inflamed.

Problems with shortened and tight psoas and piriformis muscles, weak abdominal and longissimus/erector spinae muscles and stressed quadratus lumborum muscles are very common occurrences in people who have desk jobs. As with the upper body problems associated with the Desk Distortion Posture, the one way to counteract these painful disorders is through the use of exercises and stretches laid out in this book.

The Legs

When you sit for a good portion of your day, the muscles in your legs lose their strength and become tight.

In most people the hamstring muscle group is the primary muscle in the legs that gets tight and/or painful. Because this muscle attaches to your pelvic bone, when this muscle is chronically tight, low back pain can result.

The hamstring muscles run from the bottom of the pelvis down the back of your leg and attach to your lower leg bones just below your knee joint. Your hamstrings are responsible for bending your knee and assisting in straightening up your back when you are bent forward at the hips. When you sit for an extended period of time with your knees bent, the hamstring muscles tend to become very tight and to lose strength. Tight hamstring muscles are not only uncomfortable, but they increase stress in the low back by restricting the normal movement of the pelvis, and they increase stress in the knees by restricting normal joint motion.

The Legs

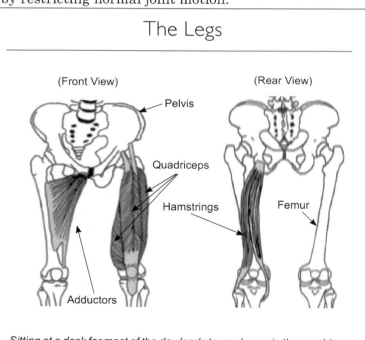

(Front View)   (Rear View)

Pelvis

Quadriceps

Hamstrings   Femur

Adductors

Sitting at a desk for most of the day leads to weakness in the quadriceps and tightness in the hamstrings. This imbalance frequently causes low back pain. For many people, as the flexibility of your hamstrings improves, your low back pain will lessen.

4

The Top 5 Desk Disasters and How to Correct Them

Sitting at a desk all day can be a disaster for your body. Part of the reason is that the lack of activity associated with working at a desk job leads to a loss of muscle strength, muscle tightness, and a loss of healthy circulation and tone. Another very common problem is that too often, your workspace is not set up correctly for your body. When your keyboard or monitor is too high or too low, your chair is not adjusted correctly, your phone is not in the correct place, or any number of other problems are present, your body is forced into an unhealthy posture. Over time, this unhealthy posture leads to chronic muscle tightness, spinal misalignments, inflammation, and pain.

In this chapter you will learn how to arrange your workspace to decrease the stress on your body while sitting at your desk. Remember, nobody sits perfectly all the time. Perfection is not the goal. The goal is to reduce your chance of injury from poor body mechanics so you can live a pain free life style.

How To Sit Correctly

Below are four sound ergonomic recommendations that will help you maintain proper body mechanics while you sit at your desk all day:

Your Eyes

Your eyes should be about an arm's length from your computer screen, if you work at a computer, and your monitor should be adjusted so that the top one-third of the monitor screen is level with your eyes. If your monitor is adjusted too high, it will cause you to tip your head back and put additional stress on your upper neck. If your monitor is too low, it will cause your head to tip forward, placing undue stress on the muscles of your lower neck, upper back and shoulders.

It is important to adjust the lighting to minimize the amount of glare off the surface of the monitor.

Your Arms and Wrists

If you use the keyboard frequently, it is important to

keep your elbows close to your body and your wrist parallel to the keyboard. Your forearms, wrists, and hands should be aligned when keyboarding and parallel to the floor. Reduce wrist strain by avoiding extension of your wrists.

Your Head and Neck

Adjust your chair and workstation so that your head is not tilted while you work. Too many people jut their head forward while they are working on their computer. This forward head posture leads to a tremendous amount of stress on the neck and upper back. Be sure to keep your head back over your shoulders.

Your Back

Adjust your chair seat and back rest to gently fit the unique contours of your back and hips, so that you can sit comfortably and straight. Position the height of the seat so that your knees are level with your hips.

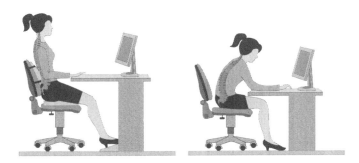

The Top Five Desk Disasters and How to Correct Them

Shrugging your shoulders, holding your head too far forward, sitting in one position, holding your mouse too far away, and slouching while you sit are five habits that wreak havoc on the body. Each of these things chronically stress the body in ways it was not designed to be stressed, which, if left unchecked, will lead to a whole host of physical problems. Let's take a look at each one of these.

Disaster One: Shrugging Your Shoulders

Shrugging your shoulders all day is a very common problem with those who work at a desk job. This is a common way that many people carry their stress. Unfortunately, chronic shoulder-shrugging leads to neck and upper back pain, headaches, as well as very tight and painful muscles. This is made worse when the height of your keyboard is not set correctly. If your keyboard is too high, you will instinctively raise your shoulders to make it easier for your hands to type on the keyboard. Here is a test that you can do to determine if you are shrugging your shoulders due to the height of your keyboard.

Self-Test

Put your left hand on your right upper trapezius muscle— the meaty area between your shoulder joint and the base of your neck—and let your right arm hang down to your side. Your right trapezius muscle should not be tight. Keeping your left hand on your right trapezius, raise up your right arm and place your hands on your keyboard as though you were about to start typing. If you feel a contraction in your trapezius when your hands are on the keyboard, then your keyboard is too high for you. The solution is to either raise your chair or lower your keyboard and repeat the test until the tightness no longer appears when your hands are on your keyboard.

Disaster Two: Holding Your Head Too Far Forward

We talked about the dangers of the forward head posture (FHP) in the previous chapter and discussed how carrying your head too far forward can lead to a whole host of chronic problems, from headaches, chronic neck and upper back pain and tightness, inflammation in the upper back and neck, as well as a loss of normal neck and head movement. This is a very common problem in people who sit all day at a desk, but it doesn't have to be so. Take this simple test to see if you are carrying your head too far forward and, if so, what you can do about it.

Self-Test

Sit at your desk in your typical sitting position. Put your hand on the back of your neck. If you feel a big dip in your neck, or it feels very tight, you are likely carrying your head too far forward. To correct this, the first step is to make sure that your vision is okay. Uncorrected vision problems are a very common cause of forward head posture as people try to bring their eyes closer to the computer screen so that they can see better. Assuming that your vision is fine, the other common culprit is a computer monitor that is either too far away or is either too high or too low. The key is to adjust the position of your computer monitor or the seat of your chair to allow your head to rest comfortably over your shoulders, instead of in front of them.

Disaster Three: Sitting In One Position ALL Day Long

Movement is necessary for a healthy body. Unfortunately, too many people spend too much of their day sitting in one position. Even though you may have found a position that is particularly comfortable for you, it is important that you change positions throughout the day. Even if you sit in a poor position for part of the day, it will not be a disaster for your body as long as you frequently switch positions.

Additionally, you can help your body even more by taking frequent breaks throughout the day. Even a two minute break once an hour where you stand up, stretch, and walk around a bit will help your body tremendously. Just avoid sitting in one position ALL day long.

Disaster Four: Holding Your Mouse Too Far Away

Just as the position of your keyboard and computer monitor have an impact on the amount of stress your body has to endure while working at a desk, so too does the position of your mouse. When you have to reach too far out when using your mouse, you are setting yourself up for a disaster with the shoulder of the arm you use to control your mouse. Having to stretch out your arm to use your mouse, you place a lot of stress on your shoulder, neck, and upper back, leading to chronic tightness, inflammation and pain.

Avoiding this problem is easy as long as you keep your mouse in the "Safe Zone." Your Safe Zone is the area on your desk that you can easily reach without having to straighten your elbow. The closer you can keep your mouse to your body, the less stress your arm and shoulder will endure when you use it.

Disaster Five: Slouching When You Sit

I saved this one for last because this is the one that almost everyone does, even though they know it is bad for them. The reason why so many people slouch is simple: gravity. When you slouch, you allow your body to slump down in a chair and let the chair hold your body up against gravity. This often times happens when we become tired or fatigued, or simply out of habit. The problem with slouching is that it places a tremendous amount of stress on the entire spine, contributes to poor posture while standing, and closes down your rib cage, restricting the full expansion of the lungs.

You can tell if you are slouching simply by paying attention to how your pelvis is positioned on the chair. When you are sitting more on your tailbone and your low back is rounded backward, then you are slouching. Changing this bad habit takes a bit of dedication, but is not difficult. The first step is just to be aware of how you are sitting. Check yourself often and if you find yourself slouching, sit up properly again. Another thing that you can do is use some props to help you retain good posture while you sit. If you sit more towards the back of the chair, a lumbar support pillow placed between your chair and the back works great. For those who find themselves sitting more towards the front of the chair, the best prop for you is an ergonomically designed seat cushion. This cushion is designed to tip your pelvis forward slightly. They look like a seat cushion with the back of the cushion higher than the front. Lastly, you will want to avoid stretching your legs out in front of you as this tends to make you slouch.

Avoiding Disaster

In this chapter you learned about the importance of proper posture while you sit at your desk as well as the five biggest disasters that commonly affect people who work at desk jobs. It is important to make the effort to reducing the stress on your body while you sit at a desk. If you follow the self-tests and the simple solutions presented in this chapter, you will feel better and reduce your neck and back stress.

5

The Daily Dozen Desk Stretches

In this chapter, you will learn the twelve most important stretches for those who work at desk jobs. I call these "The Daily Dozen Stretches." All of these can be performed while you are sitting at your desk and are pretty easy. Doing these simple stretches every day will decrease the tension in your muscles, improve your range of motion, and help you feel more comfortable as you work at your desk.

Although the demonstration pictures show the stretch being performed on one side, do both sides equally. "Time/Repetitions" represent the minimum times to get results. If one stretch feels tighter than the others, do that one more often. If you feel pain, STOP that specific stretch. Ideally, perform these stretches two times before lunch and two times after lunch.

Upper Trap Stretch

Benefits: Neck Mobility

Equipment Needed: Chair

Time / Repetitions: 15-20 Seconds on Each Side

Gently place your hand on the side of your head and gently pull to increase the stretch on your neck muscles.

Tilt your head to the side until you feel a gentle stretch.

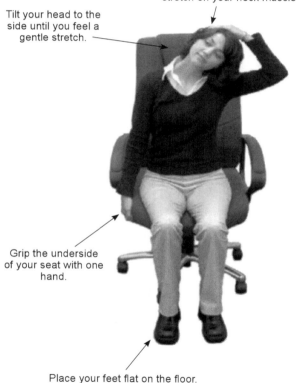

Grip the underside of your seat with one hand.

Place your feet flat on the floor.

The Levator Stretch

Benefits: Neck and Upper Back Mobility

Equipment Needed: Chair

Time / Repetitions: 15-20 Seconds on Each Side

Turn your head 45 degrees and flex your neck to the side (nose toward your elbow).

Feel the stretch on the back side of the lower neck region.

Keep your back straight.

Grip the underside back portion of your seat with one hand.

Place your feet flat on the floor.

Neck Isometrics

Benefits: Releases Neck Tension

Equipment Needed: Chair

Time / Repetitions: 10 seconds each, 4-6 Repetitions

Keep your head in a
neutral position.

Gently push head straight back
into your hands, gradually
building tension in the neck.
Hold for 10 seconds.

Place your hands on
the back of your head.

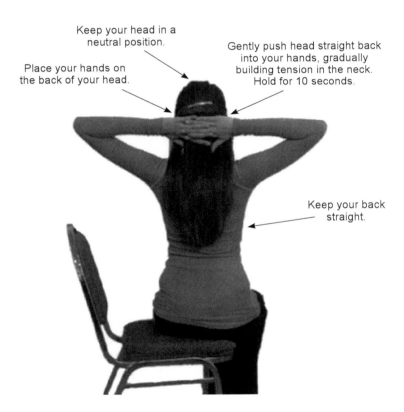

Keep your back
straight.

Place your feet flat on the floor.

Rhomboid Squeeze

Benefits: Upper Back Strength

Equipment Needed: Chair

Time / Repetitions: 10 seconds each, 5-10 Repetitions

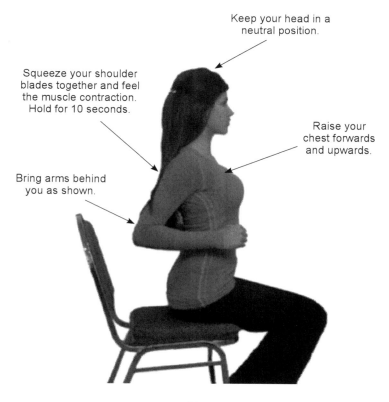

Keep your head in a neutral position.

Squeeze your shoulder blades together and feel the muscle contraction. Hold for 10 seconds.

Raise your chest forwards and upwards.

Bring arms behind you as shown.

Place your feet flat on the floor.

Neck Rolls

Benefits: Neck Mobility

Equipment Needed: Chair

Time / Repetitions: 15 Repetitions in each direction

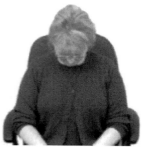
Step 1:

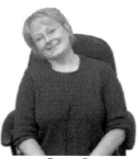
Step 2:

When doing Neck Rolls, it is important to do three things in order to properly stretch the muscles of the neck: 1) keep your shoulders level, 2) keep your face oriented forward, and 3) roll your head slowly. To be done VERY slowly.

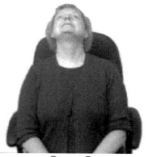
Step 3:

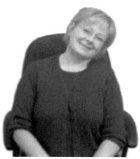
Step 4:

Hamstring Stretch

Benefits: Leg and Hip Mobility

Equipment Needed: Two Chairs

Time / Repetitions: 15-20 Seconds on Each Side, 2 Repetitions

Keep your head in a neutral position.

Keep your back straight.

Gently reach your hands out toward your feet.
Hold for 15-20 seconds.

Place one leg out in front of you.

Bend at the hips, not the lower back.

Gluteus Maximus Stretch

Benefits: Pelvis and Hip Flexibility

Equipment Needed: Chair

Time / Repetitions: 15-20 Seconds on Each Side, 2 Repetitions

Step 1:   Step 2:

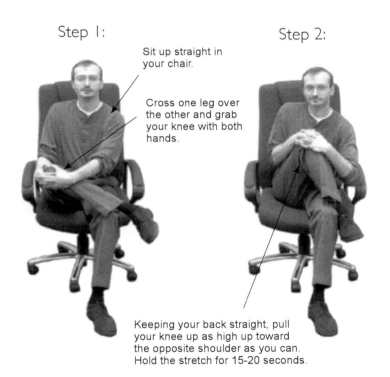

Sit up straight in
your chair.

Cross one leg over
the other and grab
your knee with both
hands.

Keeping your back straight, pull
your knee up as high up toward
the opposite shoulder as you can.
Hold the stretch for 15-20 seconds.

Quadratus Stretch

Benefits: Low Back Flexibility

Equipment Needed: Chair

Time / Repetitions: 15 Seconds on Each Side, 2 Repetitions

Turn your head in the
direction of your stretch.

Bring your arm up
over your head.

Keep your back
straight.

Lean slightly into the stretch
so that you can feel the
muscles in your low back and
side. Hold for 15 seconds.

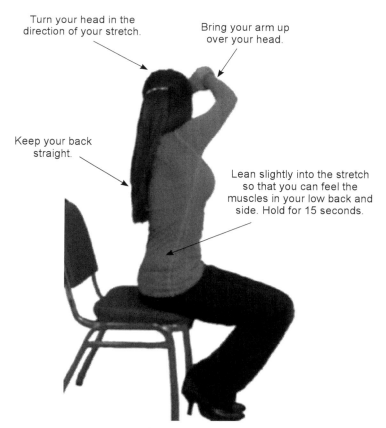

Place your feet flat on the floor.

Back Extensor Stretch

Benefits: Decrease Tension in the Low Back

Equipment Needed: Chair

Time / Repetitions: 15-20 Seconds, 2 Repetitions

Keep your head in a
neutral position.

Lift your chest upward.

Place your hands on
your hip bones and roll
your pelvis forward.
Feel the stretch in your
low back.

Place your toes on the floor and let your heels rise up.

Hip Flexor Stretch

Benefits: Low Back and Pelvis Flexibility

Equipment Needed: None

Time / Repetitions: 15-20 Seconds on Each Side, 2 Repetitions

Stand up straight and place your hands on your hips.

Push the hip of your back leg forward until you feel a stretch in the groin area.

Take a large step back with one leg and keep your back leg straight. It is normal for your heel to come up off the floor during this stretch.

Allow your front leg to bend.

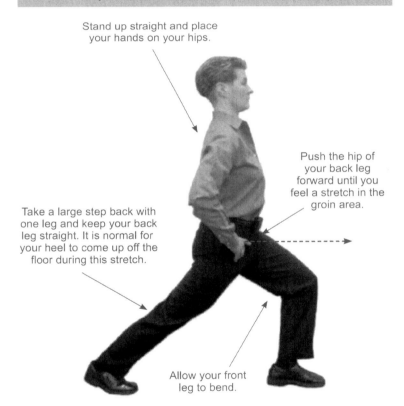

This stretch can be done while seated in a chair by scooting to the right corner of your chair and placing your right leg behind you as shown above. You would then repeat the same stretch for the left side as well.

Stick em up stretch

Benefits: reduces tension in pectoralis minor

Equipment: doorway

Time/repetitions: 10 secs   2-4 repetions.

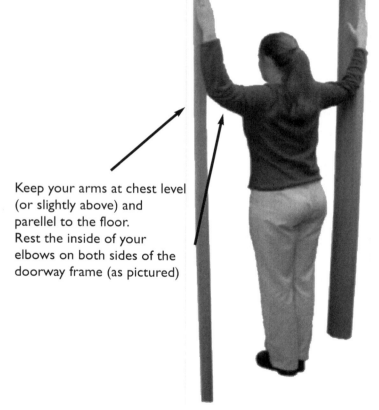

Keep your arms at chest level
(or slightly above) and
parellel to the floor.
Rest the inside of your
elbows on both sides of the
doorway frame (as pictured)

Then push your body forward till you feel a stretch
in your chest muscles.
Do not move your elbows off the doorway frame.

Get Up and Move

Benefits:	Decreases Tension and Stress
Equipment Needed;	None
Time/Reptitions:	5 Minutes/4 Times per Day

Even though these stretches will help you relieve stress and feel better while you are sitting down, it is important to remember that your body was designed to move. Taking a number of short five-minute breaks throughout the day, where you can stand up and move around, will help you immensely.

As a rule of thumb, I suggest that you stand up and go for a short walk twice before lunch and twice after lunch. This will ensure that you get at least 20 minutes of movement during your day. If you are in a work situation where you cannot get up and go for a short walk, at least make it a point of standing up and getting off your butt four times a day.

As simple as this sounds, it can make a tremendous difference in your stress level while working. If you can do more, like going for a longer walk during lunch, that's even better.

6

Body Band Exercises

For those who are a little more ambitious, up for more of a challenge, or just want some quick and effective toning, body band exercises can provide a simple and efficient way to increase your muscle strength and coordination.

In this section I will show you four body band exercises that are particularly valuable for those who work at a desk all day. They are designed to work on the primary muscle groups which frequently become stiff or injured from prolonged sitting. As with any exercise, start with a lower intensity and slowly build up the intensity. This allows your body the chance to get used to exercising and will provide the maximum benefit with the lowest chance of injury. If you have had any shoulder problems, be sure to check with your health care provider before doing these exercises.

Body Band Row

Benefits: Increase Mid-Back Tone

Equipment Needed: Chair, Body Band

Time/Repetitions: 15-20 Repetitions

Keep your head in a
neutral position.

Keeping your elbows close
to your sides, pull your hands
backward to feel the tension
in the middle of your back.

Place the band around
your knees.

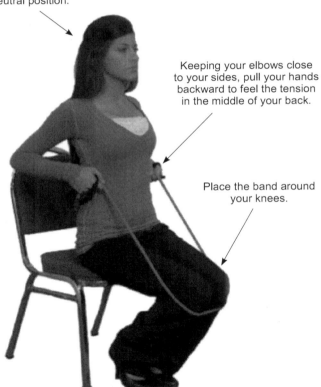

Body Band Lats

Benefits:	Increase Mid-Back Tone
Equipment Needed:	Chair, Body Band
Time / Repetitions:	15-20 Repetitions

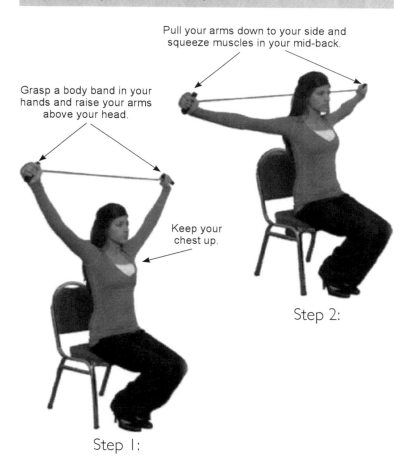

Pull your arms down to your side and squeeze muscles in your mid-back.

Grasp a body band in your hands and raise your arms above your head.

Keep your chest up.

Step 2:

Step 1:

Shoulder External Rotation

Benefits: Shoulder Mobility

Equipment Needed: Chair, Body Band

Time/Repetitions: 15-20 Repetitions

Rotate your shoulder so that your palm faces
forward. Keep your elbow bent as shown.
Then slowly return to starting position.

Secure one end of the body
band to your foot and grasp
the other end with your hand.

Keep your
chest up.

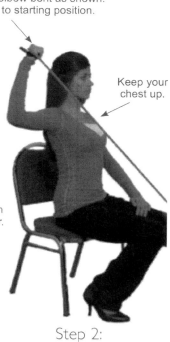

Face your palm
toward the floor.

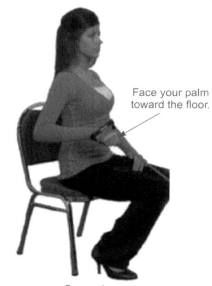

Step 2:

Step 1:

Around the clock stretch

Benefits: chest opener	
Equipment: Body band	
Time/repetitions: twice before lunch & twice after lunch.	

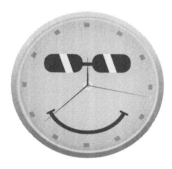

If you choose to do only one body body band exerecise
this is the one —
It's quick, effective and easy!
Hold the bands in front of you at various positions
"around the clock" and pull the bands at each end.
You will feel a stretch in your chest and slightly in your
shoulders and upper back.

7

Basic Lifestyle Enhancements

Although this chapter is not specifically about "Sitting Fit", it is about "Being Fit". It's an added bonus chapter that I believe can benefit you greatly if applied.

Chiropractic Care

This is my opportunity to tell you about what I do. In a later section, "Patients Speak," you will understand why I added this to the "lifestyle enhancement" chapter.

Yes, chiropractic care is about bones and posture, but is also about function and lifestyle. While exercise moves your bones and muscles in a general sense, chiropractic moves specific bones that are not moving properly or are out of place. For example, if someone constantly tilts their head to the right all day to view their computer, their muscles and joints will be stressed on the right side.

The word "chiropractic" comes from the Greek words cheir (hand) and praxis (action) and literally means "done by hand." Instead of prescribing drugs or performing surgeries, chiropractors use manual treatments of the spine and joints, exercise therapy, massage, trigger point therapy and lifestyle changes to improve one's health.

When you have a physical problem (i.e. a pinched nerve), you need a physical solution. When you have a chemical problem (i.e. diabetes), you need a chemical solution.

Like conventional medicine, chiropractic is based upon scientific principles of (1) diagnosis through testing and empirical observation and (2) treatment based upon the practitioner's rigorous training and clinical experience.

Chiropractic Treatment

Stretching and exercise will help to counteract the effects of poor posture, but over time the daily stress of poor posture will cause joints to "lock up." You may notice this at first as a feeling as though your neck is "a little stuck." Over time, pain and stiffness will continue to worsen. To make matters worse, when the bones in your neck are stuck or out of alignment, it causes the joints and tissues to wear out prematurely, just like a misaligned tire on your car will wear out faster than a properly aligned one.

Spinal adjustments to correct misalignments are what makes doctors of chiropractic unique in comparison with any other type of health care professional. The term "adjustment" refers to the specific manipulation chiropractors apply to vertebrae that have abnormal movement patterns or fail to function normally. The objective of the chiropractic treatment is to restore normal joint function.

Daily Exercise

According to the US Surgeon General's Report on Physical Activity and Health, regular physical activity:

- *Improves your chances of living longer and living healthier.*
- *Helps to protect you from developing heart disease.*
- *Helps to lower blood pressure and serum cholesterol.*
- *Decreases your risk of developing certain kinds of cancers.*
- *Improves bone density, thereby reducing osteoporosis.*
- *Helps to relieve pain in those suffering from arthritis.*
- *Helps to control or prevent Type II diabetes.*
- *Improves mood and relieves stress.*
- *Helps to maintain a healthy body weight.*

In their landmark book entitled Biomarkers, medical researchers Dr. William Evans and Dr. Irwin Rosenberg identified ten characteristic changes that occur as we age, including: a loss of muscle mass, a decrease in strength, a decrease in basal metabolic rate, a decrease in aerobic capacity, an increase in blood pressure, a loss of normal insulin action, a decrease in circulating HDL to total cholesterol ratio, a loss of bone density and a decreased ability to control your body temperature. Each one of these measures of physical health tends to decline as we age. What Evans and Rosenberg discovered is that exercise was effective in reversing every single one of these markers of aging!

How much exercise?

According to the U.S. Surgeon General and the American College of Sports Medicine, people "should get a minimum of 30 minutes of moderate-intensity physical activity most days of the week."

Drink Plenty of Water

Although most people can live for several weeks without food, most people can only live for a few days without water. Water, after oxygen, is the second most important substance for human health, making up about 75% of your total body weight. Water is a universal solvent and transport medium, and is used in just about every biological process in the human body, and because of this, without an adequate intake of water on a daily basis, our body will not be able to function properly.

Many Americans are dehydrated. One reason is that we consume far too many soft drinks, tea and coffee, which have a diuretic effect on the body, and the other reason is simply that we don't drink enough pure, clean water. Why is this a problem?

Water is used by your body for a whole host of important functions, such as cleansing toxins out of your body, keeping your joints and spinal discs healthy, helping your kidneys function efficiently and regulating body temperature, as well as making sure that all of the tissues in your body can heal properly and perform the necessary functions for life.

How Much Water Should You Drink?

Although everyone is different, there are two basic rules of thumb about how much water you should drink. One rule of thumb is that you should drink half of your body weight in ounces of water. For example, if you weigh 160 pounds, you should drink at least 80 oz. of water – or ten 8 oz. glasses. If you weight 200 pounds, you should drink at least 100 oz. – or about three quarts of water every day. This may sound like a lot of water, but once you get into the habit of carrying water with you and drinking it throughout the day, you will be surprised how easy it really is to consume the right amount of water.

The other rule of thumb is to drink enough water for your urine to run clear. This is the more popular approach for athletes whose daily activity may change considerably from one day to another. Because exercise increases your body's demand for water, it may be necessary to adjust how much you are drinking day-to-day, based on how much and how intensely you exercise.

Whichever way you decide will work best for you, it is important that you make drinking plenty of water part of your daily routine.

Ten Reasons To Drink More Water:

You know that drinking water is good for you, but did you know that every system in your body depends on water? Here are 10 reasons why drinking water is good for you and why you should make drinking plenty of water part of your daily routine.

1. Get healthy skin. Drinking water moisturizes your skin from the inside out. Water is essential to maintaining elasticity and suppleness and helps prevent dryness.

2. Lose weight. Increased water consumption can help you control weight by preventing you from confusing hunger with thirst. Water will also keep your body systems, including metabolism and digestion, working properly and give you the energy (and hydration) necessary for exercise.

3. Flush toxins. By helping to flush toxins, appropriate water intake lessens the burden on your kidneys and liver.

4. Reduce your risk of a heart attack. Researchers

at Loma Linda University in California studied more than 20,000 healthy men and women and found that people who drink more than five glasses of water a day were less likely to die from a heart attack or heart disease than those who drank fewer than two glasses a day.

5. Cushion and lube your joints and muscles. Water makes up a large part of the fluid that lubricates and cushions your joints and muscles. Drinking water before, during, and after exercise can also help reduce muscle cramping and premature fatigue.

6. Stay regular. Water helps prevent constipation by adding fluid to the colon and bulk to stools, making bowel movements softer and easier to pass.

7. Stay hydrated, get energized, and be alert. On average, most adults lose about 10 cups of fluid a day through sweating, exhaling, urinating, and bowel movements. Even minor dehydration can cause impaired concentration, headaches, irritability, and fatigue.

8. Regulate your body temperature. Perspiration is your body's natural mechanism to control body temperature. And to sweat, you need plenty of water.

9. Reduce your risk of disease and infection. Water can help prevent kidney stones and reduce your chances of getting bladder, kidney, and urinary tract infections. One study found that women who drank more than five glasses of water a day had a risk of colon cancer that was 45 percent less than those who drank two or fewer glasses a day.

10. Get well. The traditional prescription to "drink plenty of fluids" when you're sick still holds strong. Water can help control a fever, replace lost fluids, and thin out mucus.

Take a Multivitamin

The Journal of the American Medical Association in 2002, announced that all adults should take a vitamin supplement to help prevent a number of chronic diseases. In today's world, we are exposed to a lot of stresses that increase our body's need for vitamins and minerals. We are exposed to a constant man-made electromagnetic field from powerlines and cell phones, we eat highly processed foods that often contain artificial colors, flavors and preservatives, many of us don't get enough exercise, and we are under emotional stress at work and at home.

In order to stay healthy, we need to give our body some help. That's where supplements come in. Supplements help to ensure that your body gets all of the extra vitamins, minerals, phytonutrients and probiotics necessary to function the way it should.

Vitamins and Minerals

Following the Second World War, chemical manufacturers were sitting on huge stockpiles of phosphates and nitrates that were initially intended for use in explosives. They discovered that when they spread these same phosphates and nitrates on the soil where plants were growing, the plants grew bigger and looked healthier. Thus began the boom of the fertilizer industry.

The problem with modern fertilizers is that they don't replace soil trace minerals, such as chromium, zinc and copper, as do cow manure and other natural fertilizers. Over time, these trace minerals become more and more depleted from the soil and, consequently, our food supply becomes more depleted as well. The bottom line is that in order to get enough trace minerals in our diet to at least meet the minimum RDAs, it is necessary to take a good quality supplement.

In addition to improving your overall health, vitamins and minerals – especially the antioxidants – have been shown to decrease your risk of several diseases, such as heart disease and cancer.

How to Select a Good Multivitamin

All vitamin supplements are not created equal. Supplements are just like anything else – there are some good ones out there and a whole lot of supplements that are not as good.

What is a good quality multivitamin? I shy away from promoting any particular brand, but I can say that you usually get what you pay for. If you buy a cheap quality vitamin and your body is not digesting it all, you may think your body is getting all the nutrients in the vitamin, but what you are really getting is expensive urine.

One way to find out how digestible (bioavailability) a vitamin will be is to do a simple experiment. Place the vitamin in a bowl of vinegar. The acidity of the vinegar is close to the acidity of your stomach. If most of the vitamin does not dissolve in the vinegar after 20 minutes, it is probably not being absorbed well by the body.

Avoid Excess Sugar

There are a ton of books about why excess sugar is bad for you. The keyword here is "excess." Your diet needs to have some sugar in it. Unfortunately, most people just intake too much of it. Most people think of eating sugar (i.e.: a candy bar). However many times we *drink* more sugar than we eat. Do you drink any of the following on a daily basis?

- *A Starbucks Venti Café Latte contains 22 grams of sugar*
- *A 12 oz. can of Red Bull contains 39 grams of sugar*
- *A 20 oz. Snapple Lemon Ice Tea contains 57.5 grams of sugar*
- *A 20 ounce botle of coca-cola contains 67.5 grams of sugar*

High levels of sugar intake is very unhealthy and contributes to obesity, Type II diabetes, heart disease due to elevated triglycerides, kidney stones, dental cavities, chronic tiredness and reactive hypoglycemia. Decreasing your sugar intake is as simple as avoiding foods and beverages which are high in refined sugars. Read labels! When you purchase sweetened food, look for products that are sweetened with fruit juice or stevia, rather than sugar or high-fructose corn syrup.

Avoid Excess Hydrogenated Oils

Did you know that margarine is actually made from corn oil? That's right, the oil that is probably sitting in a clear plastic bottle in your cupboard right now is the very same oil that is used to make margarine. The process of turning corn oil is called hydrogenation. As the name suggests, hydrogenation is the process of adding hydrogen to the oil to thicken the consistency.

The problem with hydrogenation is that it changes the chemistry of the oil and introduces what are called "trans fats." Trans fats are a form of artificial fat that is created by the hydrogenation process and are not normally found in natural foods. The process is used to make an oil more solid. This provides a longer shelf-life in baked products and a certain kind of mouth watering texture to foods.

Unfortunately, they are very unhealthy and contribute to a variety of problems, such as an increased risk of heart disease and stroke. Trans fats cause a significant lowering of HDL (good) cholesterol and a significant increase in LDL (bad) cholesterol.

Some of the more common sources of hydrogenated oils in the diet include fatty foods, such as margarine and deep fried foods, but are also present in cookies, cakes, crackers, and bread.

You should get in the habit of reading labels to see what is in the foods you consume. By simply avoiding foods that contain hydrogenated oils, you can cut your consumption of trans fats almost completely. Since hydrogenated oils are only found in processed foods, avoiding them will nudge you toward a more natural diet – an added bonus!

Control Your Thoughts

A simple, but powerful story which illustrates the power of our thoughts, which was written by Mac Anderson, depicts the fact that we consciously choose our thoughts. The story goes like this: A Native American boy was talking with his grandfather. "What do you think about the world situation?" he asked. The grandfather replied, "I feel like there are two wolves fighting in my heart. One is full of anger and hatred; the other is full of love, forgiveness, and peace." "Which one will win?" asked the boy. To which the grandfather answered, "The one which I feed."

Do a self check on your 'thought life'. Is it full of anger and hatred, or is it full of love, forgiveness and peace? Does it need minor adjusting? Perhaps major adjusting? You may not be able to control all of life's circumstances, but you can control your thought process towards it.

Get Positive!

Just as negative emotions can weaken the body's resistance, positive emotions can strengthen it, or at least allow it to function normally. The simple act of deciding to be happier and focusing on the positive will improve your health. In fact, this phenomenon of your thoughts affecting your physical health is so strong that all medical studies have to be designed with it in mind. Researchers call this phenomenon 'the placebo effect.'

Many people believe that the term "placebo effect" means that the effect is only imagined – that it is not real. But this couldn't be further from the truth. Medical studies have to include a control group – people who receive placebos instead of the medicine being studied – because the simple act of people making the decision to take action to improve their health leads to measurable physical improvement in their condition. To determine how much of an effect a particular medicine had, the researchers have to take the measured change in the group who underwent the particular therapy and subtract out the amount of change seen in the placebo group. Otherwise, there is no way to know whether a particular treatment was beneficial or whether it was merely the change in attitude in the study subjects that made the difference. In many instances, the placebo effect turns out to be stronger than the treatment itself!

When it comes to 'controling our thoughts', Saint Paul says it best, "Whatever is true, whatever is worthy of respect whatever is just, whatever is pure, whatever is lovely, whatever is commendable, if something is excellent or praiseworthy, *think* about these things."

Five Minutes of Solitude

Modern life is full of pressure, stress and frustration. Worrying about your job security, being overworked, driving in rush-hour traffic, arguing with your spouse — all these create stress. According to a recent survey by the American Psychology Association, fifty-four percent of Americans are concerned about the level of stress in their everyday lives and two-thirds of Americans say they are likely to seek help for stress.

One way to combat the stresses of life is to regularly "replenish" your soul.

Steven Covey, in his book "The Seven Habits of Highly Effective People," has a great story about this principle. He calls it "sharpening your saw." It is about replenishing yourself. In this story, you are supposed to imagine that you come upon someone in the woods working feverishly to saw down a tree.

"What are you doing?" you ask.

"Can't you see?" comes the impatient reply, "I'm sawing down this tree."

"You look exhausted!" you exclaim. "How long have you been at it?"

"Over five hours" he returns, "and I am beat! This is hard work."

"Well why don't you take a break for a few minutes and sharpen that saw?" you inquire. "I'm sure it would go a lot faster."

"I don't have time to sharpen the saw," the man says emphatically. "I'm too busy sawing!"

In this busy life in which we all live, don't forget to take the time to sharpen your saw regularly. Replenishing your soul will strengthen you so you will be more effective, efficient and happy. Everyone is different as to what replenishes them and how often they need to sharpen their saw.

Some examples of sharpening your saw are: reading, being alone in nature, praying, meditation, exercising, watching a movie, traveling, etc. Find what feeds your soul and feed it regularly! Take time with the intention of replenishing yourself. So when life gives you trees to saw down, you will be able to do it effectively, efficiently and with joy in your heart.

My Closing Thoughts —

I hope you enjoyed this journey with me and that you will Sit Fit and Be Fit more regularly. I don't expect anyone to apply all the principles in this book all at once. So use this as a reference book. Apply what "jumped out at you" while reading this book NOW. Then revisit this book and apply some other principles later on. Also don't forget to teach your friends and co-workers how to Sit Fit and Be Fit as well.

Lastly, if you enjoyed this book, please send me an email with your comments at drcheryl14141@gmail.com

Wishing you many years of good health,

Dr. Cheryl Gottesfeld, D.C.

8

Patients Speak

"Dr. G is the Best! No more aching back ... or migraines!"

"So much relief in such a short time! Thanks!"

"Dr G is an excellent diagnostician and clinician! She's been taking care of me and my patients for ten years and she's a warm person."

"The five-minute miracle" – 53 year old basketball player"

"I've tried other chiropractors, but Dr. Cheryl is the best!!"

"My yard work is getting done ... Thanks, Dr G"

"Dr. G has kept me out of surgery for five years! The Best!"

"Walking is good. Walking pain free is even better."

"Dr. Cheryl is fantastic. I haven't been this relaxed in my neck in two years or more. She's wonderful."

"Dr. G is the 'pain buster', you're the best."

"Dr. Cheryl's treatments are a cornerstone of my health management plan!"

"I am free at last of pain."

"Our family has had many years of good health thanks to Cheryl!"

"Dr. Gottesfeld is a mainstay in my total physical and mental well being, we need more people like her!"

"Dr. G is an angel in my life. She has been blessed with knowing her true calling in life – to use her gifted hands to help others. She is completely trustworthy and truly cares for you and your health."

"From my first visit I felt R-E-L-I-E-F You are the best!!"

"Wow! Just a few cracks and suddenly the pain is gone– No more pressure – feel taller – like there's more space in between each vertebra – Thanks so much."

"I drive an hour to have Cheryl 'keep me going' at 66, I feel great."

"Straightens me right up ... Restores physical and mental clarity. Helps the quality of my life."

"You have helped both of us so much."

"Nothing like a good chiropractor! It's nice to function normally!"

9

References

1. *Brunswic M. Ergonomics of seat design. Physiol, 70 (2): 40–43, 1984*

2. *During J, Goudfrooij H, Keensen W, et al. Toward standards for posture: Postural characteristics of the lower back system in normal and pathologic conditions. Spine, 10 (1): 83–7, 1985*

3. *Keegan JJ. Alterations of the lumbar curve related to posture and seating. J Bone Joint Surg, 35 (3): 589–603, 1953*

4. *McKenzie RA. The lumbar spine: mechanical diagnosis and therapy. Waikanae, NZ: Spinal Publications LTD, 1981*

5. *Magora A. Investigation of the relation between low back pain and occupation. Scand J Rehab Med, 5: 186–190, 1975*

6. *Kelsy JL. An epidemiological study of acute herniated lumbar vertebral discs. Rheumatol and Rehab 14: 144–159, 1975*

7. *Schoberth H. Sitzhalten. Sitzschaden. Sitzmobel. Berlin: Springer, 1962. Referred to in AC Mandal. The seated man (Homo sedens): The seated work position. Theory and Practice. Applied Ergo 12 (1): 19–26, 1981*

8. *Mandal AC. The correct height of school furniture. Physiol 70 (2): 48–53, 1984*

9. *Cailliet R. Neck and arm pain. Philadelphia: FA Davis Co., 1981*

10. *Mayo Clinic Health Letter, Vol 18 (3), March 2000*

11. *Gore DR, Sepic SB, Gardner GM. Roentgenographic findings of the cervical spine in asymptomatic people. Spine, 6: 591–694, 1986*

To Order Copies of This Book

1. Order at Amazon.com

2. Order at Barnes and Nobles (BN.com)

3. Download e-book from your Kindle, Nook, Sony E-reader, ipad, ipod.

4. Contact our office at:
   Dr. Cheryl Gottesfeld, D.C.
   4141 North Henderson Road, # 14
   Arlington, VA 22203
   Phone: (703) 276-1891
   www.ArlingtonChiropractor.com